YOUR KNOWLEDGE HAS VALUE

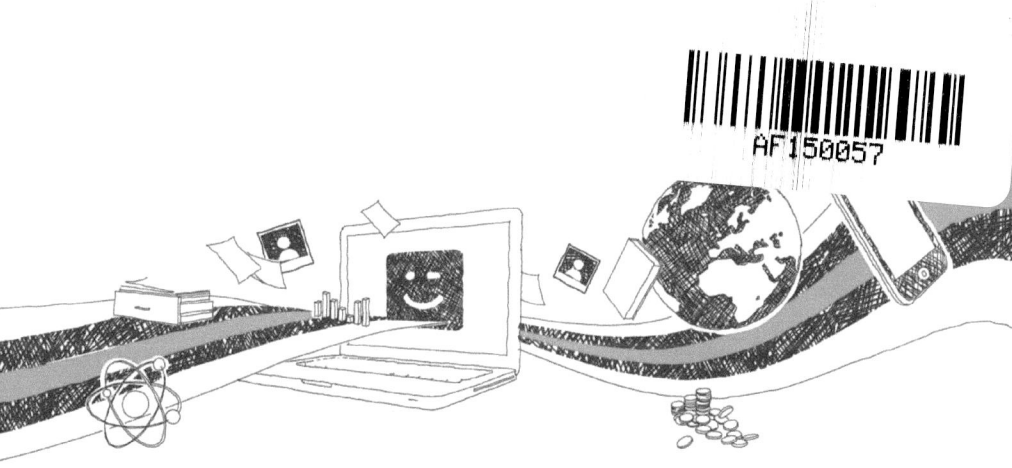

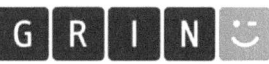

Bibliographic information published by the German National Library:

The German National Library lists this publication in the National Bibliography; detailed bibliographic data are available on the Internet at http://dnb.dnb.de .

Imprint:

Copyright © 2016 GRIN Verlag, Open Publishing GmbH
Print and binding: Books on Demand GmbH, Norderstedt Germany
ISBN: 9783668278387

This book at GRIN:

http://www.grin.com/en/e-book/338105/the-association-between-circulating-levels-of-myeloperoxidase-and-type

Perez Kisakye Katambala

The association between circulating levels of myeloper-oxidase and type 2 diabetes in the Malmö diet and cancer cohort. An Assessment

GRIN Publishing

GRIN - Your knowledge has value

Since its foundation in 1998, GRIN has specialized in publishing academic texts by students, college teachers and other academics as e-book and printed book. The website www.grin.com is an ideal platform for presenting term papers, final papers, scientific essays, dissertations and specialist books.

Assessing the association between circulating levels of myeloperoxidase, a marker of chronic inflammation, and type 2 diabetes in the Malmö diet and cancer cohort

June 2016

Abstract

Background

Chronic inflammation is suggested to play an important role in the pathogenesis of many chronic conditions. Chronic inflammatory biomarker Myeloperoxidase (MPO) has been reported in several studies that have investigated its role in cardiopulmonary events. However, there are limited studies that investigated its relationship with type 2 diabetes.

Objectives

To investigate the relationship between plasma MPO concentration and lifestyle and socioeconomic factors and incident type 2 diabetes mellitus in the Malmö diet and cancer cohort (MDC).

Method

This was a prospective cohort study of 4544 participants drawn from MDC cardiovascular sub-cohort, with no type 2 diabetes at baseline between 1991 and 1996. Plasma MPO concentration were measured using Olink CVD kit. The cox proportional hazard regression analysis was used to determine the relationship of plasma MPO concentration with incident type 2 diabetes.

Results

Age, obesity, education level, Hb1Ac, plasma insulin, and plasma glucose were associated with MPO concentration. There was significant association between plasma MPO concentration with the risk of incident type 2 diabetes, crude hazard ratio (HR) 1.67 (95% CI 1.36–2.05) for higher plasma MPO concentration (quartile 4) compared with the lowest (quartile 1). This association persisted after further adjustment for age, sex, smoking, education level and BMI with a slight reduction in the risk, HR 1.48 (95% CI 1.2 – 1.82) for MPO quartile 4.

Conclusion

Our results suggest that age, obesity, education level, Hb1Ac, plasma insulin, and plasma glucose, are predictors of the chronic inflammatory biomarker plasma MPO concentration, which in turn are associated with risk of type 2 diabetes mellitus among females and males who participated in the MDC cardiovascular cohort. Before MPO can be used as a measure for preclinical type 2 diabetes or insulin resistance, its pathophysiological role needs to be further studied.

Table of contents

List of abbreviations

ACS	Acute coronary syndrome
BMI	Body Mass Index
CAD	Coronary Artery Disease
CVD	Cardiovascular Disease
DNA	Deoxyribose nucleic acid
EDTA	Ethylenediaminetetra acetic acid
EGIR	European Group of insulin study of insulin resistance
ELISA	Enzyme Linked Immunosorbent Assay
Hb1Ac	Glycosylated haemoglobin
HOMA	Homeostasis model assessment
HOMA-IR	Homeostasis model assessment of insulin resistance
IL-6	Interleukin 6
ITN-6	Interferon 6
LDL	Low density lipoprotein
LTA	Leisure time activity
LTPA	Leisure time physical activity
LU	Lund University
MDC	Malmo diet and cancer cohort
MHR	Malmo HbA1c register
MMP-9	Matrix metalloprotease 9
MPO	Myeloperoxidase
NDR	National diabetes register
NK	Natural Killer cells
OGTT	Oral glucose tolerance test
PCR	Polymerised chain reaction
PEA	Proximity extension assay
PMNs	Polymorphonuclear neutrophils
ROS	Reactive oxidative stress
RT	Real time
SPSS	Statistical package for social scientists
TNFα	Tumour necrosis factor α

WHO   World Health Organisation

INTRODUCTION

According to the World Health Organisation (WHO), the estimated global diabetes prevalence in 2014 was 9% among adults 18 years or older and in 2012 diabetic attributable deaths were estimated at 1.5 million. More than 80% of these deaths occur in low and middle income countries and it was projected that it will be the 7th leading lone cause of death in 2030(1). Globally type 2 diabetes comprises 90% of the total diabetic patient population; type 2 diabetes is attributed to obesity and sedentary lifestyle(1). Unabated diabetes is associated with poor prognosis, resulting from morbidity and mortality which compromises the quality of life. It requires high costs to control diabetes and treatment of its acute and chronic complications(2). All diabetes prevalence in Sweden was estimated to be 6.8% in 2013 and projected to be 10.4% by the year 2050 affecting over 940000 individuals(3).

Diabetes is a chronic metabolic disorder that occurs when the pancreas does not produce insulin or when the body cannot effectively utilize the insulin produced(4). Insulin is a hormone required for the glucose in blood to be transformed into energy by the body cells. Type 2 diabetes is characterized by insulin resistance by target organs and less insulin production by the pancreas.

Inflammation is a protective response which involves host cells, blood vessels and proteins with primary intent to remove cause of injury, eradicate dead body cells and tissue and again start off the process of repair. It is a localized protective response to trauma or microbial invasion that destroys, dilutes or shields off the injurious agent and the injured tissue(5). The process is normally controlled and self-limited. It is characterised by redness, hotness, swelling, loss of function and pain often localized to the affected area. This process can occur in response to mechanical trauma, toxins and neoplasia. Excessive inflammation may cause abnormal recognition of host tissue as foreign or chronic inflammatory process may lead to inflammatory diseases such as type 2 diabetes, atherosclerosis and Alzheimer's disease and syndromes such as rheumatic fever and rheumatic heart disease(5). The polymorphonuclear neutrophils (PMNs) and macrophages constitute part of the defensive white blood cells and are wide spread throughout the human body. They have a major role in innate immunity, their programmed cell death and removal is imperative in effective resolution of acute inflammation(6). However, these cells have azurophilic granules which contain an enzyme Myeloperoxidase (MPO) which is a haem protein released into extracellular fluid during inflammatory processes and is said to be associated with bacterial destruction and oxidative tissue injury(6,7). During inflammation there is activation of PMNs, a process referred to as respiratory burst, which leads to production and release of superoxide, hydrogen peroxide and other reactive oxygen species (ROS) which are toxic to microbes(8). The enzyme MPO catalyses the reaction between hydrogen peroxide and free chloride ions forming hypochlorous acid which is over fifty times more toxic than hydrogen peroxide to bacteria(8). It is believed that MPO plays a central role in killing fungi, protozoa, viruses, tumour cells, natural killer (NK) cells, red blood cells and blood platelets(8). Overproduction of ROS causes oxidative stress, hyperglycaemic states and creates an imbalance in glucose metabolism (9,10). Several studies have supported the hypothesis that chronic subclinical inflammation may be associated with insulin resistance and precede the development of clinically overt type 2 diabetes (11).

In a matched cohort study, it was found out that chronic organ specific and multisystem inflammatory conditions were associated with high risk of incidence type 2 diabetes(12). Recent findings show that concentrations of acute-phase response markers and mediators of inflammation cytokines such as Tumour Necrosis Factor α (TNFα) and interleukin-6 (ITN-6) are raised in people with type 2 diabetes(13). In a prospective multicentre case-control study, obesity was found to be characterized with chronic subclinical inflammation(14) and elevated concentration of MPO was observed in adipose tissue of animal models and humans. This enzyme plays an important role in the initiation and progression of chronic conditions such a Coronary Artery Disease (CAD)(14). It has been observed that MPO in blood is higher in patients with acute coronary syndrome (ACS) and it is not specific only for cardiac diseases, since activation of neutrophils and macrophages can be caused by several other conditions including infections (7). Recent findings suggest that elevated MPO blood levels among patients with ACS have poor prognostic outcomes(15). It has been highlighted that rising MPO levels among diabetic patients is greatly associated with progression of atherosclerosis(16). However, studies examining the association between MPO levels and risk of type 2 diabetes are lacking. Similarly, MPO could be both a direct and indirect early biomarker of systemic inflammation(17).

Public Health Relevance

Inflammation is a normal physiological process which enhances recovery and tissue repair after injury. If left unabated it can predispose one to getting future type 2 diabetes mellitus and its associated costs.

Aim of the study

To assess the association between chronic inflammation and incident type 2 diabetes in the Malmö diet and cancer cohort (MDC) by analysing chronic inflammatory MPO plasma biomarker. The MDC cohort is a large prospective population study where a wide array of clinical and non-clinical investigations are conducted to answer different research questions from a Swedish perspective.

Objectives

1. To investigate the relationship between MPO concentration and lifestyle and socioeconomic, i.e., obesity, smoking, physical activity and education.

2. To investigate the relationship between plasma MPO concentration with incident type 2 diabetes mellitus.

METHOD AND MATERIALS

Study sample.

The Malmö Diet and Cancer Study (MDC) is a population-based, prospective cohort of 28449 men (born 1923-1945) and women (born 1923-1950) from Malmö, south of Sweden, who underwent baseline examinations between 1991 to 1996. At baseline, a detailed clinical examination including; dietary assessment, a self-administered questionnaire, anthropometry was done and peripheral venous blood samples drawn were archived in biological bank(18). From the main cohort, a subsample of 6,103 participants were randomly invited and accepted to participate in a sub-cohort study (MDC cardiovascular cohort). A total of 5533 accepted to participate and attended the second visit at the study screening centre and had overnight fasting venous blood samples drawn for plasma separation. Participants had a number of test measurements done in their blood sample including; fasting blood glucose, plasma insulin, and erythrocyte glycosylated haemoglobin (Hb1Ac) among others.

We excluded 368 of these subjects from the study due to incomplete clinical data, while another 307 subjects did not have plasma available. The remaining 4865 subjects whose plasma samples were sent for analysis, 123 subjects were further excluded because the analysis of their plasma samples did not pass the internal quality control for the biomarker analysis. The remaining 4742 subjects were followed from baseline examination until first event, we excluded 196 with prevalent type 2 diabetes and other 2 more, who had missing MPO results, the remaining 4544 were considered for analysis. Prevalent type 2 diabetes was defined at baseline as; self-reported according to the questionnaire (had a response 'Yes' to the question 'Do you have diabetes'), use of anti-diabetic medication or basing on records from national and regional registers(19).

Consent

All participants gave written consent at enrolment before any study procedures were done and the original study obtained the ethical approval from the Regional Ethical Review Board, Lund, Sweden (LU 51/90).

Identification of incident diabetes

Our outcome measure was incident type 2 diabetes mellitus and was defined as diagnosis made after date of enrolment during follow-up, from baseline until first diagnosis (that is until December 31, 2014) and were identified through national and regional registers. Type 2 diabetes mellitus cases were identified from the Malmo Hb1Ac Register (MHR) at Clinical chemistry, the Swedish National Diabetes Register (NDR), the Swedish Hospital Discharge Register, the Nationwide Drug Prescription register and the Scania region Diabetes 2000 Register(19). For an incident case to be entered in the NDR and Diabetes 2000 register, it required a physician diagnosis after a thorough assessment following the diagnostic criterion of; taking the participants' fasting plasma glucose concentration with values of equal to $7.0mmolL^{-1}$ or greater which is identical with fasting whole blood glucose of $6.1mmolL^{-1}$ or more(19).

Furthermore, incident type 2 diabetes mellitus cases were identified through reassessment of the cohort. The selection criteria identifying incident cases was either by considering; (i) responses given in the questionnaire, (ii) use of antidiabetic drugs, (iii) fasting plasma glucose and oral glucose tolerance test (OGTT). The OGTT was done by participants having 30g oral load of glucose and after 120 minutes, had whole blood test for glucose concentration, any value equal to $7.0mmolL^{-1}$ or more was considered to be glucose intolerant(20). At least one independent source of registered type 2 diabetes mellitus was a confirmed case.

Biochemical MPO Analysis

Proseek® Multiplex CVD I 96×96 was the reagent kit that was used to measure 92 CVD - related human protein biomarkers, including MPO, simultaneously in plasma frozen at negative 80°C until analysis. A volume of 45mls of venous blood was collected from study participants at baseline and their ethylenediaminetetra acetic acid (EDTA) – plasma concentration of MPO was measured using Proseek Multiplex method, an immunological technique used in biomarker discovery. This technique uses antibodies like in the Enzyme Linked Immunosorbent Assay (ELISA) and the output results are by real time (RT) polymerised chain reaction (PCR). The Proseek reagents are based on a Proximity Extension Assay technology (PEA), where oligonucleotide labelled antibody probe pairs are allowed to bind to their respective target present in the sample in this case MPO biomarker. A PCR reporter sequence was formed by a proximity dependent DNA polymerization event and was subsequently detected and quantified using real-time PCR. The data output was for relative quantification. Therefore, for MPO the data obtained was not of absolute values (pg/ml) but instead described differences in MPO levels between samples and groups.

Measurements and definition of variables

Participants invited at the first visit and consented, were given a questionnaire that was collected at study visit two and was checked for completeness. It assessed for highest education attained categorised as; elementary, primary and secondary, upper secondary, further education without a degree and university degree. The smoking habit was categorised as; never smoked, former smokers, current smoker (regular or occasional smoker). The leisure-time physical activity index was obtained by use of leisure time activity (LTA) questionnaire which included questions on 17 predefined activities and open ended questions(21). The leisure activity comprised of the sum total of all activities adjusted for intensity and was categorised as low for lower quartile, moderate for quartile 2, high for quartile 3 and very high for upper quartile.

Participants' weight (kg) was taken with balance-beam scale and their standing up height measured using standiometer in centimetres later converted to meters without shoes by two trained nurses (19,22), with participants putting on light clothing and their supine position blood pressure (mmHg) was measured 10 minutes after resting(23). Waist circumference (cm) was taken at the level of the umbilicus with a tape measure. The body mass index (BMI)(kg/m^2) was computed using the standard formula of weight (kg)/square of height(m).

Plasma insulin was measured using nonspecific radioimmunoassay(23) set at detection limit of 3mIU/L with intra and inter-assay coefficients of variations 5 and 8% respectively and blood glucose was measured using hexokinase technique(21). Erythrocyte HbA1c was determined by ion exchange chromatography technique, using the Swedish Mono-S standardization with reference values of 3.9 - 5.3 % for non-diabetics(19).

Homeostasis model assessment (HOMA) a measure of insulin resistance was according to the European Group of insulin study of insulin resistance (EGIR) and was determined by the model; [fasting insulin (mIU/L) x fasting blood glucose]/22.5(23).

Statistical Analysis

Statistical analysis was done using IBM – SSPS package, version 22.0 for Windows. Normal distribution of MPO was done using frequency distribution across the sample and reported using a histogram and plasma insulin was widely dispersed and transformed logarithmically for statistical analysis. We used two sided tests with statistical levels of significance assumed when P<0.05. We categorized MPO concentrations into quartiles and calculated descriptive statistics of the sample including mean and standard deviation. The association between MPO quartiles and continuous variables (age, BMI, plasma glucose, plasma insulin, HOMA-IR and HbA1c) were analysed using general linear model. Crude association between MPO quartiles and categorical variables (sex, smoking, education level and LTPA) were analysed using chi square test (table 1).

Cox regression was used to calculate hazard ratios at 95% confidence intervals (CI) to investigate association of MPO quartiles and incident type 2 diabetes mellitus with time of follow-up as the time variable. In the basic model we adjusted for age and sex. In a multivariate model, we adjusted for; age, sex, smoking and education. In another multivariate model, adjusted for; age, sex, smoking, education and BMI. We also performed a model adjusted for age, sex, smoking, education, BMI and HbA1c.

RESULTS

The total sample comprised of 4544 participants and their plasma was analysed for MPO inflammatory biomarker and were composed of 2756(60.7%) females and 1788(39.3%) males. Figure 1 a histogram showing a frequency distribution of MPO across the population. The mean MPO concentration was 3.46(standard deviation of 0.35). Table 1 describes the participant characteristics presented in the MPO four quartiles. It shows that age, BMI, plasma glucose, plasma insulin, HOMA-IR and Hb1Ac all have an increasing trend across the MPO quartiles from Quartile 1 to Quartile 4. MPO concentration decreases with increasing education levels; the majority in the 4th quartile of MPO had elementary education 555(27.0%) as compared with those with university education 76 (22.4%) in the same quartile. Table 2 shows the distribution of incident type 2 diabetes across the four MPO quartiles with the largest number of 228 cases in quartile 4 with the shortest person years of 20083 as compared with the rest. To investigate the association between MPO and the risk of type 2 diabetes mellitus we ran a Cox regression analysis (table 2) and calculated the crude hazard ratio (HR) (crude model). We found an increased risk with higher MPO concentrations that is, crude HR 1.67 (95% CI 1.36–2.05) for MPO quartile 4 compared with quartile 1. Further adjustment for age, sex, smoking, education, BMI and Hb1Ac (Multivariate model ^{c}) slightly reduced the risk HR 1.41 (95% CI 1.14–1.73), for MPO quartiles 4.

DISCUSSION

This was a prospective cohort study on the association between plasma MPO concentrations and incident type 2 diabetes mellitus. Our findings from analysis suggest that plasma MPO concentration are associated with the risk of incident type 2 diabetes mellitus suggesting how important chronic inflammation is associated with the risk of incident type 2 diabetes mellitus. Our results also revealed an association between MPO concentration and age, BMI, plasma glucose, natural logarithm of plasma insulin, HOMA-IR and Hb1A.

In our study, we found that the elderly had higher concentrations of plasma MPO, as compared with the younger counterparts. An explanation to this could be that as one grows there is a tendency of getting several inflammatory conditions. Similarly, our findings are consistent with a study done in China where elderly patients had significantly higher concentrations of MPO as compared with the young counterparts(24), it was also found out that ageing is associated with oxidative stress with low grade inflammation independent of any disease condition(25).

We found that BMI, a marker of obesity, significantly increased with higher plasma MPO concentration. Similar observations were revealed in a study which aimed at assessing levels of MPO among obese volunteers with or without inflammation(26). This could be fronted to justify why obesity is a risk factor for incident type 2 diabetes mellitus. However, clear mechanisms underpinning the process of low grade inflammation among obese subjects is still lacking.

To determine an individuals' historical blood glucose concentration, HbA1c test is routinely done for this purpose. In our study we found out that Hb1Ac significantly increased with rising MPO concentration and hence the risk of incident type 2 diabetes mellitus. However, in a study which included 40 poorly controlled glycaemic type 2 diabetes mellitus patients, 30 with good control and 31 non diabetic patients, it was found that MPO concentration decreased with rising Hb1Ac across all groups(27). Notably, in a study which investigated association between MPO and blood pressure by assessing effects of hyperglycaemia and oxidative stress, it was found out that plasma MPO concentration increased with rising plasma glucose(28) and another study also had similar findings(29). The explanation for these observations for both Hb1Ac and plasma glucose rising with MPO concentration is still unclear.

This study noted a pattern of increasing plasma insulin across the MPO quartiles being significantly higher in the fourth quartile. In a large cross sectional community-based Framingham study of 2,002 non diabetic subjects, it was found that similarly the plasma MPO concentration was high among subjects who had higher plasma insulin concentration, a measure of insulin resistance(30). This shows that several participants in our sample were having insulin resistance a preclinical feature of type 2 diabetes mellitus and there is a possibility of delaying or preventing incident type 2 diabetes mellitus endpoint if they consider re-modification of their lifestyle. These findings are of clinical importance and can be used in teasing out preclinical type 2 diabetes mellitus and can offer a basis in routine clinical management.

In this study we found that smoking was not significantly associated with MPO concentration (P=0.06); however, we noted that 27.1% were smokers in the fourth compared with 24.7% in the first and 22.5% in the second quartile   . In a study which assessed the association of genetic variation with susceptibility for cigarette smoke-induced neutrophilia, it was found that short term exposure to cigarette smoking caused airway inflammation in humans and animal models, and showed a positive correlation with MPO levels(31). In another study which assessed serum levels of MPO from 4,677 subjects who had mild to moderate airflow limitation in the Lung Health Study(32), it was found that MPO concentration was significantly higher among smokers. In our study it is possible that significant effects of smoking with plasma MPO concentration were masked by the small number of smokers in our sample. We therefore do not refute the possibilities of significant association between plasma MPO concentration with smoking.

Our study revealed no significant effects of leisure time physical activity on MPO levels. Carrie. P, et al reported on a study that examined the effects of intensive physical activity on human athletes and rat blood neutrophil degeneration, where it was found that MPO levels increased in both human athletes and animal models after exercise(33). This effect was found to be temporal where the MPO levels normalized after a few hours after resting(33). Another study which investigated the relationship between maximal exercise, induced increases in serum IL-6 (interleukin-6), MPO and MMP-9 (matrix metalloprotease-9) concentrations(34), found that maximal exercises augmented the increase in inflammatory biomarkers including MPO contrarily to what we found out. However, the validity of these findings can be refuted wholly or in part on the basis of the small study sample and the demographic characteristics of participants that was studied. In another study that assessed the association of MPO, non-oxidised LDL (low density lipoproteins) with leisure time physical activity, it was found out that MPO concentration may reduce among individuals who are more active as compared with their counterparts(35). It is possible that in our study by the time participants were bled they had their leisure time physical activity in more than three hours similarly as reported by Carrie. P and there was no neutrophil degeneration to cause changes in plasma MPO concentration.

We also revealed that individuals' education level was associated with plasma MPO concentration levels. There is no direct scientific link between someone's education level and plasma MPO concentration but it can be asserted that the higher the education level someone attains, the less the risk of higher plasma MPO concentration attributed to risk exposure and hence type 2 diabetes endpoint. This can be attributed to the nature of occupation, knowledge base about the type 2 diabetes mellitus which enhances avoidance of possible risk factors education can offer. It can be assumed as well that the time individuals spend in education institutions also limits their exposure to possible occupational risks that can enhance higher plasma concentrations of MPO and hence type 2 diabetes mellitus endpoint.

Strengths and Limitations of the study

The strengths of our study were: large study population who had completed their questionnaires and had their blood sample pass the internal biochemistry quality control for MPO analysis. The other strength was that type 2 diabetes mellitus diagnosis was recorded after MPO levels were measured which reduced the possibility of selection bias.

The most important limitation of our study is that participants did not have follow up plasma MPO concentration analysis for comparison. As a result, we cannot determine whether those who had elevated plasma MPO concentration at baseline maintained this status quo until incident type 2 diabetes mellitus endpoint.

Clinical implications

We believe that the results of our study could offer clinical implications in the future. Our study revealed that, by far; age, BMI, Plasma insulin, HOMA-IR, HbA1c and education level are predictors of MPO levels and thereby risk factors of incident type 2 diabetes mellitus. We underpin the importance of having lifestyle behaviours under control that are associated with elevation of BMI for primordial prevention of type 2 diabetes mellitus. We have noted that elevation of plasma MPO concentration is associated with incident type 2 diabetes mellitus and could be a possible target of novel treatment of chronic inflammatory conditions. Because higher plasma MPO concentration could play a direct or indirect role in causal pathway of incident type 2 diabetes mellitus, we suggest further inquiry into this pathogenesis.

CONCLUSION

In conclusion, our results suggest that age, obesity, education level, Hb1Ac, plasma insulin, and plasma glucose, are predictors of the chronic inflammatory biomarker plasma MPO concentration, which in turn are associated with the risk of type 2 diabetes mellitus among females and males who participated in the MDC cardiovascular cohort. Before MPO can be used as a measure for preclinical type 2 diabetes or insulin resistance, its pathophysiological role needs to be further studied.

REFERENCES

(1) WHO. Diabetes Fact sheet N°312. 2015; Available at: http://www.who.int/mediacentre/factsheets/fs312/en/. Accessed February 23, 2016.

(2) Nogueira Cortez D, Afonso Reis I, Silva Souza DA, Lopes Macedo MM, de CT. Complications and the time of diagnosis of diabetes mellitus in primary care. ACTA PAUL ENFERMAGEM 2015 05;28(3):250-255 6p.

(3) Andersson T, Ahlbom A, Carlsson S. Diabetes Prevalence in Sweden at Present and Projections for Year 2050. PLoS One 2015;10(11):e0143084. doi:10.1371/journal.pone.0143084.

(4) International Diabetes Federation. What is diabetes? 2016; Available at: http://www.idf.org/worlddiabetesday/toolkit/gp/what-is-diabetes. Accessed April/23, 2016.

(5) Douglas T, Fearon, Barton F,Haynes, Carl N editors. INFLAMMATION Basic principles and clinical correlates. 3rd ed. Philadelphia: Lippincott Williams & Wilkins; 1999.

(6) El Kebir D, Jozsef L, Pan W, Filep JG. Myeloperoxidase delays neutrophil apoptosis through CD11b/CD18 integrins and prolongs inflammation. Circ Res 2008 Aug 15;103(4):352-359.

(7) Loria V, Dato I, Graziani F, Biasucci LM. Myeloperoxidase: a new biomarker of inflammation in ischemic heart disease and acute coronary syndromes. Mediators Inflamm 2008;2008:135625.

(8) eBioscience. Human MPO Instant ELISA. 2015; Available at: http://www.ebioscience.com/human-mpo-instant-elisa-kit.htm. Accessed 03/09, 2016.

(9) Fatani SH, Babakr AT, NourEldin EM, Almarzouki AA. Lipid peroxidation is associated with poor control of type-2 diabetes mellitus. Diabetes Metab Syndr 2016 Jan 14.

(10) Ntimbane T, Krishnamoorthy P, Huot C, Legault L, Jacob SV, Brunet S, et al. Oxidative stress and cystic fibrosis-related diabetes: a pilot study in children. J Cyst Fibros 2008 Sep;7(5):373-384.

(11) Pitsavos C, Tampourlou M, Panagiotakos DB, Skoumas Y, Chrysohoou C, Nomikos T, et al. Association Between Low-Grade Systemic Inflammation and Type 2 Diabetes Mellitus Among Men and Women from the ATTICA Study. Rev Diabet Stud 2007 07;4(2):98-104.

(12) Dregan A, Charlton J, Chowienczyk P, Gulliford MC. Chronic Inflammatory Disorders and Risk of Type 2 Diabetes Mellitus, Coronary Heart Disease, and Stroke: A Population-Based Cohort Study. Circulation 2014 June 26.

(13) Schmidt MI, Duncan BB, Sharrett AR, Lindberg G, Savage PJ, Offenbacher S, et al. Markers of inflammation and prediction of diabetes mellitus in adults (Atherosclerosis Risk in Communities study): a cohort study. Lancet 1999 05/15;353(9165):1649-1652.

(14) Olza J, Aguilera CM, Gil-Campos M, Leis R, Bueno G, Martinez-Jimenez MD, et al. Myeloperoxidase is an early biomarker of inflammation and cardiovascular risk in prepubertal obese children. Diabetes Care 2012 Nov;35(11):2373-2376.

(15) Kolodziej AR, Campbell CL, Charnigo R, Twerenbold R, Mueller C, Ziada KM, et al. Abstract 221: Prognostic Role of elevated Myeloperoxidase in Patients with Acute Coronary Syndrome: A Systemic Review and Meta-Analysis. Circulation Research 2014 July 18;115(Suppl 1):A221-A221.

(16) Kataoka Y, Shao M, Wolski K, Uno K, Puri R, Murat Tuzcu E, et al. Myeloperoxidase levels predict accelerated progression of coronary atherosclerosis in diabetic patients: insights from intravascular ultrasound. Atherosclerosis 2014 Feb;232(2):377-383.

(17) Andelid K, Bake B, Rak S, Linden A, Rosengren A, Ekberg-Jansson A. Myeloperoxidase as a marker of increasing systemic inflammation in smokers without severe airway symptoms. Respir Med 2007 May;101(5):888-895.

(18) Manjer J, Carlsson S, Elmstahl S, Gullberg B, Janzon L, Lindstrom M, et al. The Malmo Diet and Cancer Study: representativity, cancer incidence and mortality in participants and non-participants. Eur J Cancer Prev 2001 Dec;10(6):489-499.

(19) Engstrom G, Smith JG, Persson M, Nilsson PM, Melander O, Hedblad B. Red cell distribution width, haemoglobin A1c and incidence of diabetes mellitus. J Intern Med 2014 Aug;276(2):174-183.

(20) Berglund G, Nilsson P, Eriksson K-, Nilsson J-, Hedblad B, Kristenson H, et al. Long-term outcome of the Malmö Preventive Project: mortality and cardiovascular morbidity. J Intern Med 2000;247(1):19-29.

(21) Nilsson PM, Engstrom G, Hedblad B. The metabolic syndrome and incidence of cardiovascular disease in non-diabetic subjects--a population-based study comparing three different definitions. Diabet Med 2007 May;24(5):464-472.

(22) Mattisson I, Wirfalt E, Aronsson CA, Wallstrom P, Sonestedt E, Gullberg B, et al. Misreporting of energy: prevalence, characteristics of misreporters and influence on observed risk estimates in the Malmo Diet and Cancer cohort. Br J Nutr 2005 Nov;94(5):832-842.

(23) Hedblad B, Nilsson P, Engström G, Berglund G, Janzon L. Insulin resistance in non-diabetic subjects is associated with increased incidence of myocardial infarction and death. Diabetic Med 2002;19(6):470-475.

(24) Fan Q, Chen L, Cheng S, Li F, Lau WB, Wang LF, et al. Aging Aggravates Nitrate-Mediated ROS/RNS Changes. Oxid Med Cell Longev 2014;2014:10.1155/2014/376313.

(25) Petersen KS, Smith C. Ageing-Associated Oxidative Stress and Inflammation Are Alleviated by Products from Grapes. Oxid Med Cell Longev 2016;2016:6236309.

(26) Borato DC, Parabocz GC, Ribas JT, Netto HP, Erdmann FC, Wiecheteck LD, et al. Biomarkers in Obesity: Serum Myeloperoxidase and Traditional Cardiac Risk Parameters. Exp Clin Endocrinol Diabetes 2016 Jan;124(1):49-54.

(27) Unubol M, Yavasoglu I, Kacar F, Guney E, Omurlu IK, Ture M, et al. Relationship between glycemic control and histochemical myeloperoxidase activity in neutrophils in patients with type 2 diabetes. Diabetol Metab Syndr 2015;7:10.1186/s13098-015-0115-3.

(28) Van der Zwan LP, Scheffer PG, Dekker JM, Stehouwer CD, Heine RJ, Teerlink T. Hyperglycemia and oxidative stress strengthen the association between myeloperoxidase and blood pressure. Hypertension 2010 Jun;55(6):1366-1372.

(29) Zhang X, Dong L, Wang Q, Xie X. The relationship between fasting plasma glucose and MPO in patients with acute coronary syndrome. BMC Cardiovasc Disord 2015;15:10.1186/s12872-015-0088-z.

(30) Meigs JB, Larson MG, Fox CS, Keaney JF,Jr, Vasan RS, Benjamin EJ. Association of oxidative stress, insulin resistance, and diabetes risk phenotypes: the Framingham Offspring Study. Diabetes Care 2007 Oct;30(10):2529-2535.

(31) Pouwels SD, Heijink IH, Brouwer U, Gras R, den Boef LE, Boezen HM, et al. Genetic variation associates with susceptibility for cigarette smoke-induced neutrophilia in mice. Am J Physiol Lung Cell Mol Physiol 2015 Apr 1;308(7):L693-709.

(32) Park HY, Man SF, Tashkin D, Wise RA, Connett JE, Anthonisen NA, et al. The relation of serum myeloperoxidase to disease progression and mortality in patients with chronic obstructive pulmonary disease (COPD). PLoS One 2013 Apr 18;8(4):e61315.

(33) Saylor C,P editor. Weight Loss, Exercise and Health Research. 1st ed. New York: Nova Science Publishers, Inc; 2006.

(34) Reihmane D, Jurka A, Tretjakovs P. The relationship between maximal exercise-induced increases in serum IL-6, MPO and MMP-9 concentrations. Scand J Immunol 2012 Aug;76(2):188-192.

(35) Autenrieth C,S., Emeny R,T., Herder,Christian, DÃ¶ring,Angela, Peters,Annette, Koenig,Wolfgang, et al. Myeloperoxidase, but not oxidized LDL, is associated with leisure-time physical activity: Results from the MONICA/KORA Augsburg Studies 1984–1995. Atherosclerosis 2011;219(2):774-7. doi: 10.1016/j.atherosclerosis.2011.07.125. Epub 2011 Aug 5.

List of figures and tables

Figure 1. Histogram showing the distribution of MPO across the study sample

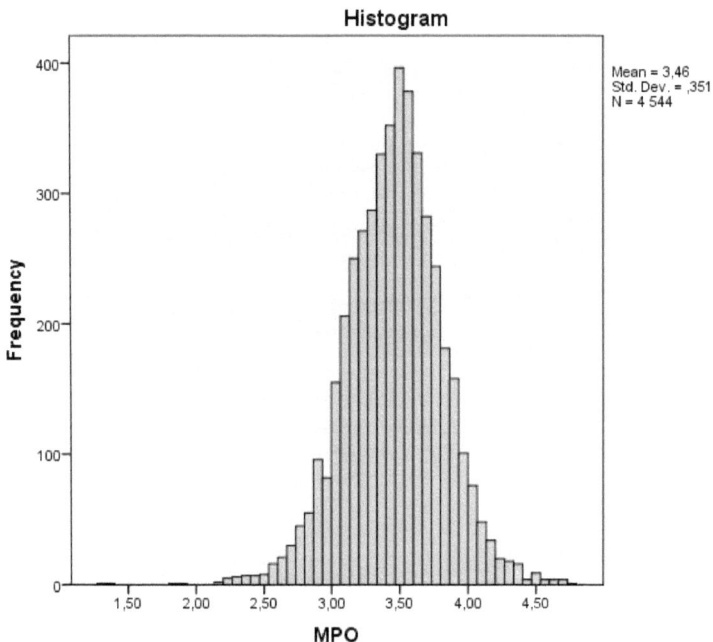

Table 1. Participant characteristics presented in the four MPO quartiles

Variables	MPO Quartiles				P-value
	1	2	3	4	
	(n=1160)	(n=1141)	(n=1121)	(n=1122)	
	Mean (SE)				
Age, years	56.9 (0.2)	57.1 (0.2)	57.7 (0.2)	58.1 (0.2)	<0.001
BMI, kg/m^2	25.2 (0.1)	25.4 (0.1)	25.8 (0.1)	26.0 (0.1)	<0.001
Plasma glucose, mmol/L	5.59 (0.02)	5.64 (0.02)	5.70 (0.02)	5.67 (0.02)	0.03
*Ln-plasma insulin, pmol/L	3.62 (0.02)	3.65 (0.02)	3.69 (0.02)	3.70 (0.02)	<0.001
HOMA-IR	1.52 (0.04)	1.59 (0.04)	1.66 (0.04)	1.73 (0.04)	<0.001
HbA1c (%)	4.76 (0.01)	4.78 (0.01)	4.82 (0.01)	4.85 (0.01)	<0.001
	N (%)				
Sex					0.12
Male	488(27.3)	425(23.8)	440(24.6)	435(24.3)	
Female	672(24.4)	716(26.0)	681(24.7)	687(24.9)	
Smoking					0.06
Smokers	298(24.7)	271(22.5)	310(25.7)	326(27.1)	
Ex-smokers	385(25.9)	393(26.4)	372(25.0)	336(22.6)	
Never smokers	476(25.8)	477(25.8)	436(23.6)	459(24.8)	
Education					<0.001
Elementary	467(22.7)	513(25.0)	520(25.3)	555(27.0)	
Primary and secondary	317(26.0)	314(25.8)	301(24.7)	287(23.5)	
Upper secondary	98(25.1)	104(26.6)	97(24.8)	92(23.5)	
Further education without a degree	96(28.3)	78(23.0)	89(26.3)	76(22.4)	
University degree	180(34.0)	131(24.7)	111(20.9)	108(20.4)	
Leisure-time physical activity					0.57
Low	276(24.8)	283(25.4)	266(23.9)	289(25.9)	
Moderate	276(24.5)	290(25.7)	298(26.4)	263(23.3)	
High	293(25.9)	294(26.0)	273(24.1)	272(24.0)	
Very high	311(27.4)	268(23.6)	273(24.1)	283(24.9)	

All results are expressed as numbers (N) and percentages (%) for MPO quartiles 1, 2, 3 and 4. BMI, Body mass index; Ln Plasma insulin, Natural logarithm of Plasma insulin, HOMA-IR, Homeostasis model assessment of insulin resistance. *Natural logarithm of plasma insulin was considered due to the wide dispersion of the absolute values of plasma insulin.

Table 2: Association (hazard ratios and 95% CI) between MPO and risk of type 2
diabetes

	MPO Quartiles				
	1 (n=1160)	2 (n=1141)	3 (n=1121)	4 (n=1122)	P-value
Cases/person-years	150/22240	184/21515	203/20167	228/20083	
Crude model	1.00	1.25 (1.00-1.54)	1.47 (1.19-1.82)	1.67 (1.36-2.05)	<0.001
Basic model	1.00	1.27 (1.02-1.57)	1.48 (1.20-1.82)	1.67 (1.36-2.05)	<0.001
Multivariate model [a]	1.00	1.26 (1.01-1.56)	1.45 (1.18-1.79)	1.64 (1.34-2.02)	<0.001
Multivariate model [b]	1.00	1.24 (1.00-1.54)	1.37 (1.11-1.69)	1.48 (1.20-1.82)	<0.001
Multivariate model [c]	1.00	1.23 (0.99-1.52)	1.22 (0.98-1.52)	1.41 (1.14-1.73)	0.002

Crude model unadjusted

Basic model Adjusted for age and sex

Multivariate model [a] Adjusted for age, sex, smoking, education

Multivariate model [b] Adjusted for age, sex, smoking, education, BMI

Multivariate model [c] Adjusted for age, sex, smoking, education, BMI, HbA1c

APPENDIX

POPULAR SCIENCE SUMMARY

When our bodies are challenged with factors from outside or from within, we hurt and we perceive this as pain, the affected area turns red, swells, feels hot at times may cause fever and loss of function of the affected area because any manipulation worsens the pain. This condition is termed to as inflammation. This is a normal natural way how our bodies restore back to normal function by removing underlying cause and enhance repair of the damaged body cells. However, when this condition is prolonged it can cause lifelong illnesses.

We investigated the possibility of whether chronic inflammation is associated with the risk of future development of adult form of diabetes, a type which does not occur during pregnancy. We investigated 4544 individuals who had no diabetes when they entered the study between 1991 and 1996. In their blood, a marker of chronic inflammation (myeloperoxidase) was measured. We identified individuals who had developed adult form of diabetes by 31 December 2014 from different registries. In our analysis, we determined that those individuals who had high blood concentration of the chronic inflammatory marker, had a 41% higher risk of developing adult form of diabetes compared with those individuals with low blood concentration.

To delay or reduce this risk we recommend all individuals involved to treat any form of inflammation early or if where possible to avoid getting one, as it will save one from costs associated with treating adult form of diabetes and its complications.

ACKNOWLEDGEMENT

I would like to thank the Swedish government through the Swedish Institute for the generous offer of my scholarship which enabled me to attend this invaluable course in one of the best universities in the world, it would not have been possible without your support. My special thanks and acknowledgement go to the program administration and all my lecturers who have guided me throughout my academic tenure in the MPH program all your concerted efforts have helped achieve my study objective right from the start.

I convey special thanks to my supervisor, Professor Emily Sonestedt, your guidance and patience has been invaluable throughout this project and has imparted in me values I will always draw from. To my colleagues of the year 2016, you are all great, you made learning in discussion groups very interesting with a global blend, sharing experiences generously by far made the program more robust and practical, and I am confident that we are ready to improve global health.

Special thanks go to my lovely family; my wife Angela, daughters Alicia and Nicole you have been by my side throughout my study tenure far away from home. The great Mugoya Family you are special, you endlessly encouraged me to push and hung on until this program was brought to completion, thank you. Maria Kappel Therese, I convey special thanks to you for your indelible encouragement and emotional support. Above all I would like to thank the Almighty God for His endless guidance, favour, protection and providence all throughout my life and education career.

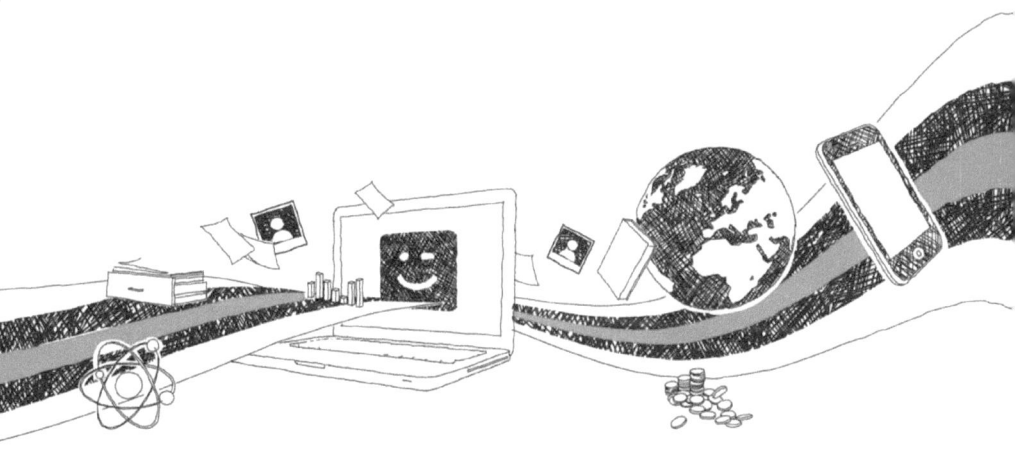
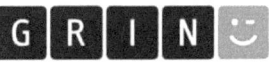